SHONICA JAQUES, MSN, RN

Pacemakers Demystified

A Quick Guide to Your Heart's New Best Friend

First published by Red Dirt Publishing 2023

Copyright © 2023 by Shonica Jaques, MSN, RN

All rights reserved. No part of this publication may be reproduced, stored or transmitted in any form or by any means, electronic, mechanical, photocopying, recording, scanning, or otherwise without written permission from the publisher. It is illegal to copy this book, post it to a website, or distribute it by any other means without permission.

Shonica Jaques, MSN, RN asserts the moral right to be identified as the author of this work.

Shonica Jaques, MSN, RN has no responsibility for the persistence or accuracy of URLs for external or third-party Internet Websites referred to in this publication and does not guarantee that any content on such Websites is, or will remain, accurate or appropriate.

Designations used by companies to distinguish their products are often claimed as trademarks. All brand names and product names used in this book and on its cover are trade names, service marks, trademarks and registered trademarks of their respective owners. The publishers and the book are not associated with any product or vendor mentioned in this book. None of the companies referenced within the book have endorsed the book.

First edition

*This book was professionally typeset on Reedsy.
Find out more at reedsy.com*

Two of the most important gifts God has given me are the sweet, sassy, smart, and full-of-life boys I call my sons, Noah and Knox. Through all of the ups and downs, the frustrations and joys, and the plain chaos of our lives together, my deepest hope and prayer for you both is that you know that Jesus didn't die in vain; God has BIG, BIG plans for you to prosper and be loved more than you could ever hope, dream or imagine. I mess up a lot, babies, but God never does.
Love you. Mean It.
Mom

"Each of you should use whatever gift you have received to serve others, as faithful stewards of God's grace in its various forms" 1 Peter 4:10.

Contents

Preface ii
1. Introduction 1
2. History of the Implantable Cardiac Device 3
3. Anatomy of the Heart 8
4. Indications for a Pacemaker 11
5. Implant Procedure 13
6. After The Implant 16
7. Device Interrogation 18
8. Living with a Pacemaker 21
9. Remote Monitoring 24
10. Conclusion 27
11. FAQs 29
12. References 33

About the Author 35

Preface

I never saw myself tickling people's hearts (as a call it) and operating a machine that can change the pace of a person's heartbeat. Here I am though, rocking it.

I had no idea what I was getting myself into when I clawed my way through nursing school fighting depression at the same time. The devil saw something in me a long time ago and has been trying to hold me back with depression for over 20 years now. I'm not gonna say he hasn't won some battles along the way, because he has. I have given up a time or two. I have lacked a WHOLE LOT of motivation at times. I have lived in survival mode for many, many years "circling the city walls" as Joshua did at Jericho because I know that I know that I know that Jesus didn't die in vain. God had and still has BIG plans for me. He didn't and won't give up on me, so I am going to keep on swimming as long as I need to to reach my goals and His plans for my life. And here I am. By the grace of God ONLY, here I am.

This book is purely a solution to my patients' main problem which is a lack of knowledge about their new pacemakers. I have been a device clinic nurse for 2 years, and it didn't take very long for me to realize there was a very real issue for patients with newly implanted devices and even patients who have had their devices for a couple of years but have never been able to find the resources they need to be educated about this amazing and very complicated device they now carry around inside of their bodies.

I didn't realize until I had been a nurse for quite some time that my dad's ability to talk to just about anyone was a trait he passed along to me. As a nurse, I have realized the importance of being educated so that I can pass along that information to my patients. Whether its cardiac device nursing, operating room nursing, or plain old med-surge nursing, our patients depend on us and look to us to calm their fears. They expect us to know what we are talking about and to be able to verbalize it to them so they understand. This is a gift I consider to have been given. Thus, I share my knowledge with you, my long-distance patient, and I hope that my knowledge comes across clearly and helps you to live your best life with your new (or old) pacemaker.

1

Introduction

Lub, dub. Lub, dub. Lub, dub. Those are the sounds of your heart. As a nurse, they are one of the first things you learn how to assess, the sounds of the life-sustaining organ in your chest: your heart. It is one of the organs that doesn't need your purposeful thought to use, and thank God it doesn't! Can you imagine having to think about making your heart beat every few seconds? What else would you get done? Nothing! You'd be a slave to your heart. Instead, your brain sends it automatic instructions to keep beating in order to keep you alive. But what happens when this essential organ stops working on its own?

PACEMAKERS DEMYSTIFIED

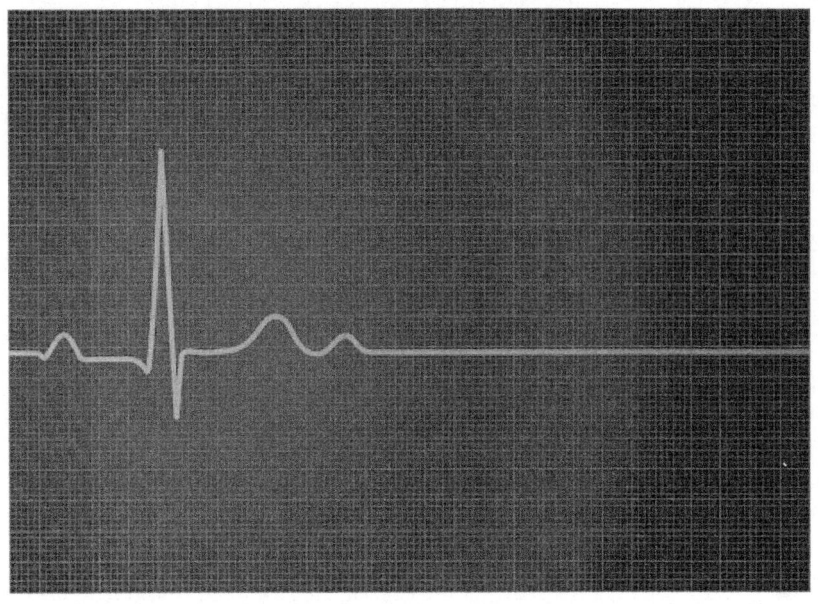

2

History of the Implantable Cardiac Device

If we were having this conversation long before 1960, the answer would be: the patient died. In 1958, a thoracic surgeon named Ake Senning "implanted myocardial electrodes and a pulse generator with a rechargeable nickel-cadmium battery" (Jeffrey & Parsonnet, 1998). Senning, along with Swedish engineer, Rune Elmqvist, had worked on the device over a two-year period for it to fail only a few hours after it was implanted. A second device they tried lasted six weeks before it failed. That patient received another pacemaker in 1960, and he was still living in 1998 after having had 26 pacemakers in total. Arne Larsson, who was 40 years old when he received the first pacemaker, lived to be 83 years old and died in 2001 (van Hemel & van der Wall, 2008). A variety of batteries and wires kept him alive for 43 years. It's amazing what we can do in the world of medicine!

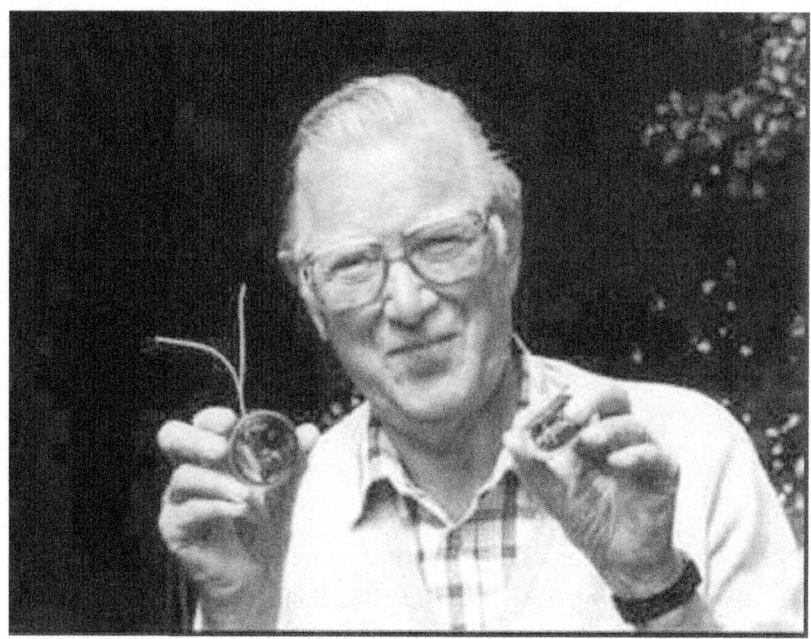

A photo of Arne Larsson holding a pacemaker similar to the first successful pacemaker placed inside of his own chest in 1958. (Morris, 2017).

Two years after Senning's first implantable device, William M. Chardack implanted the first battery-powered pacemaker with a myocardial lead (which means a wire implanted into heart tissue). His patient was a 77-year-old man who wore a football helmet on a daily basis because of the number of fainting spells he had experienced. Once he had a working pacemaker, he was able to live without fear of constantly passing out and was able to lead a normal life for 2 ½ years before he passed away. Not only were pacemakers allowing people to live longer, they were also improving the quality of their lives.

In the years to come, several other physicians worked with engineers to create numerous similar devices (Jeffrey & Parsonnet, 1998). Over the next decade, advances were made in the size of the devices, their reliability and power source, their overall ability to pace and the actual implant procedure. Though the first pacemakers were predicted to last 3-5 years, they often ceased working in much less time, or their unpredictability resulted in emergent replacement surgeries. Broken leads and erratic pacing behavior plagued these early devices. Different types of power sources were experimented with to prolong battery life and reliability including a nuclear generator option. The early batteries leaned towards utilizing much more energy than necessary to make the heart beat which led to premature depletion. Early pacemakers did not sense the patient's own intrinsic heartbeat and delivered impulses whether the heart needed them or not. What is now known as noncompetitive pacing was first introduced in the 1960s to allow the patient's own heart to beat when it could and the pacemaker to intervene only when necessary. This type of pacing was another solution presented to the ongoing battle with battery longevity.

During the same decade, the surgical procedure to implant pacemakers got an upgrade. The procedure originally used to implant pacemakers was a thoracotomy which involved a large incision to the lateral chest wall and exposure of the heart muscle. This changed in the 1960s when the transvenous approach was developed. By the mid-1960s, the field of implanting physicians expanded from just cardiothoracic surgeons to include a new breed of cardiologist known as the electrophysiologist who specialized in diagnosing and treating issues with your heart's electrical system.

The 1970s saw the acceptance of the lithium battery as the gold standard for pacemaker power sources. The chemistry of the lithium battery led to a more condensed-size pacemaker as well as the ability for the device to be hermetically sealed to prevent any body fluids from entering the device once it was implanted. These batteries depleted at a much more reliable pace which gave physicians a better chance of knowing when the device would need to be replaced, dramatically reducing the number of emergent replacement surgeries.

During the same decade, the ability to individualize treatment became mainstream with the introduction of noninvasive pacemaker programming. In the 1950s, the first generators were external, allowing physicians to alter treatment as needed. During the 1960s, treatment alteration required minor surgery. As of 1972, the next generation of pacemakers allowed for programming through the ancestors of today's external programmers. Using a magnet, the physician was able to vibrate switches inside the generator to make programming changes. These programmable changes included six pacing options and four output choices. By the end of the 1970s, multi-programmable units were invented and the ability to not only change the programming after implantation but also to communicate with the device to monitor its "stimulation rate, battery voltage and impedance, lead impedance, and the integrity of the encapsulation in the implanted device" was made available (Jeffrey & Parsonnet, 1998). The concept of dual-chamber pacing was broached but did not pick up speed until the 1980s due to the complexity of electrical circuitry needed to bring the idea to fruition which increased the size of the pacemaker as well as improved the battery's rate of depletion.

Until the introduction of the dual-chamber pacer, pacemakers only had one lead, and it was implanted into the ventricle. The invention of a lead more readily implanted into the atrium as well as new innovations in implantation methods of anchoring the electrode tip into the atrial muscle led to dual-chamber pacing becoming more of the norm in the 1980s. Having two pacing wires helped the device to emulate normal physiologic heart function. Because of this, pacemaker and battery usage could fluctuate based on the patient's own need for cardiac output. The newfound multi-functionality of pacemakers has greatly increased the variety of indications for pacemaker placement.

The 1990s saw the increasing automation of the pacemaker as

well as its self-diagnostic capabilities. The devices of the 90s were microprocessor-driven and could detect and record events based on how the physician programmed them just as they still do today. In the 2000s, cardiac resynchronization therapy (CRT), also known as biventricular pacing, was introduced to help patients with cardiomyopathy and heart failure (Aquilina, 2006). Many pacemaker-related complications are associated with the leads which have led to the invention of the leadless pacemaker. Today, 7 million people benefit from the use of an implantable cardiac device. Remote monitoring has led to better patient outcomes and earlier device malfunction detection and remote interrogation techniques have advanced to the point of automatic home checks reducing the need for clinic visits. The future may hold batteryless pacemakers (Madhavan, et al., 2017). Considering the technological advances made between 1958 and sixty-five years later, the sky is the limit as to where cardiac device engineers may take cardiac devices in the next sixty-five years.

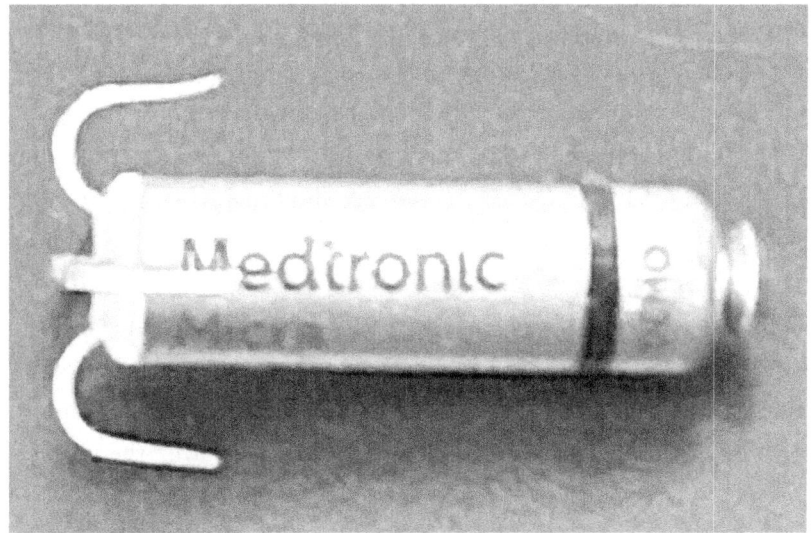

The Medtronic Micra Leadless Pacemaker

3

Anatomy of the Heart

The human heart has four chambers: two upper chambers called atria and two lower chambers called ventricles. The electrical stimulus flows through a type of cell in the heart known as the electrical conduction system. The signal starts in the sinoatrial node, or SA node, and travels along the following path: from the SA node to the atrioventricular node (AV node) to the Bundle of His along the bundle branches ending in the Purkinje fibers.

Just as in other muscles of the body, electrical impulses cause the muscles they stimulate to contract and relax. Unlike other muscles of the body that are needed to contract and relax when you need to control them to kick a soccer ball, move your arm or pick something up with your fingers, for example, the heart muscle has to work continuously. For that to happen, your brain sends signals to the autonomic nervous system which then tells the electrical system in the heart to conduct electrical impulses in a particular order and in particular timing intervals to keep the body circulating the blood it needs to take oxygen to the cells that need it without any purposeful thought from you.

The first impulse produced by the SA node (located in the right atrium) causes the atria to begin to contract. The next stop for the electrical impulse is the AV node. This bunch of cells is smaller than the SA node, and it is located in the wall between the right atria and right ventricle. Because the cluster of cells is smaller in the AV node, it transmits the signal more slowly giving the ventricles the signal to begin to contract but only after a slight delay giving them time to fill with blood from the atria. The signal then reaches the Bundle of His where it shoots through the heart muscle like a flash of lightning moving deeper into the heart muscle. Right about where the atria turn into the ventricles, the Bundle of His branches into the left and right bundle branches. These two branches carry the electrical signal into the deepest parts of the heart on both the left and right sides. As the electrical signal reaches the end of the conduction pathway, it fans out into the bottom of the heart in what looks like the shape of an upside down umbrella: the bundle of His being the handle, the bundle branches being the stem, and the Purkinje fibers being the canopy of the umbrella. As the electrical signal travels upwards along the outer edges of the heart, the ventricles squeeze the blood up and out of the heart, and a new signal begins again at the SA node.

Electrical system of the heart

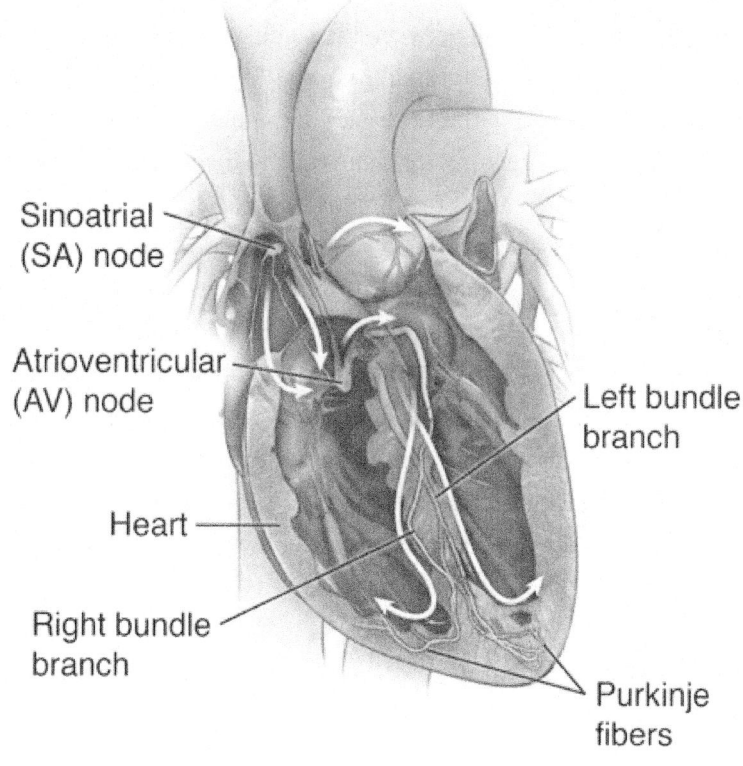

4

Indications for a Pacemaker

So, what happens when you have a broken heart? Well, depending on the problem, you either need to see a therapist or a cardiologist. More specifically, if your heart beats too fast or too slow, you need to see an electrophysiologist or EP. A healthy heart rate is between 60 and 100 beats per minute (bpm). If your heart beats slower than 60 bpm, it is called a bradycardia (brady means slow). On the other hand, if your heartbeat is greater than 100 bpm, it is referred to as a tachycardia (tachy means fast). Ongoing heart rhythms like these are known as arrhythmias (either bradyarrhythmias or tachyarrhythmias respectively).

Bradyarrhythmias occur because of problems with the electrical conduction system (see above section). Cells within the system can be damaged due to scarring or heart attack. Tachyarrhythmias often occur due to what is called re-entry. A loop of electrical activity occurs making a certain part of the heart beat faster than it normally would or out of order. This can happen in the bottom of the heart (called a ventricular tachycardia), in the top of the heart (an atrial tachycardia or supraventricular tachycardia) or at the level of the AV node.

The most common reasons, or indications, for having a pacemaker implanted are sinus node dysfunction and AV block. Sinus node dysfunction is also known as sick sinus syndrome. It is officially diagnosed when there is documented symptomatic bradycardia with frequent pauses or symptomatic bradycardia due to required drug therapy in relation to another medical condition such as hypertension. Symptomatic chronotropic incompetence occurs when your heart cannot keep your heart rate elevated where it is needed when you are engaged in physical activity or exercise. This is another indication that a pacemaker is necessary.

Sinus bradycardia with a heart rate less than 40 bpm and no clear reason for the bradycardia is also an indication for pacemaker implantation. Also included in indications are unexplained syncope or fainting and chronic heart rate less than 40 bpm even if the patient is minimally symptomatic (Dalia and Amr, 2022). Any one of the many causes for AV block which results, most commonly, in fainting are all indications for pacemaker as the lower half of the heart's electrical system does not work sufficiently or at all to push blood out into circulation throughout the body.. Severe cardiomyopathy related to systemic heart failure is an indication for cardiovascular resynchronization therapy which involves pacemaker implantation to try to synchronize both the left and right ventricles to beat at the same time for a better "squeeze" and increased blood flow circulation. This diagnosis is usually made by measurements from an echocardiogram which show left ventricular ejection fraction less than or equal to 35%. While this is not an exhaustive list, these are the most common indications for pacemaker implantation.

5

Implant Procedure

If you don't already have a pacemaker, you may be wondering what the procedure is like to have one implanted. On the day of your surgery, you will have an IV placed in your arm for IV fluids and IV medications. You will lie flat on the operating room table, and your anesthesia care provider will give you some medication to make you drowsy. You will not be completely sedated rather you will most likely drift in and out of consciousness during the procedure. Once you are drowsy, your OR team will clean the area of skin on your chest where the cardiologist or EP will be inserting the device. The rest of your body will be covered with towels and drapes to keep the area sterile.

When the physician begins, he or she will inject a local anesthetic in the skin where he will then make a 5-6 cm long incision just below your collarbone on your non-dominant side. If you have an objection to the non-dominant side being used (for example you hunt or play a sport that requires the non-dominant side of your body or non-dominant shoulder to be used more than the dominant side, this can be changed as there is no right or wrong side. You will be unable to lift anything weighing more than a gallon of milk on the chosen side, as well as, be unable to raise the arm on that side above your head for approximately

4 weeks after implant in an effort to prevent lead dislodgement or migration.

Once the incision is made, a sheath is placed into the subclavian vein to make way for the leads or wires that will be connected to your pacemaker to give your heart the electrical impulses it needs to pump blood. Using x-rays to visualize the vasculature, the cardiologist guides the leads into the correct chamber of your heart, and each lead will become embedded into the heart tissue to eventually transmit the electrical impulses when needed to the heart muscle.

At this point in the procedure, the cardiologist will test the leads to measure how much electrical current will need to be used to make the muscles contract. That measurement along with a few others are recorded and used in the programming of your generator. The physician will be working with a medical device representative from the company that manufactured the device that is being implanted to set, or program, your pacemaker specifically for the best treatment plan for you.

Once the device is programmed, the leads are attached to the generator (pacemaker). The physician creates a pocket between the skin and the chest muscle where the pacemaker will be placed. A non-dissolvable suture may be placed to hold the pacemaker in the pocket, and the original incision will then be closed with dissolvable stitches. Some doctors will then place steri-strips (small pieces of tape to hold the two sides of the incision together) while others prefer to use skin glue to ensure the incision is closed. They may also put a waterproof dressing on top of the steri-strips/skin glue to keep the area dry for the first week or two.

The entire procedure will take approximately one hour (unless you are having a biventricular pacemaker placed which is a more complicated surgery involving three leads instead of one or two.) You will have to stay overnight in the hospital, and you will require the next day to rest and recover from the procedure.

6

After The Implant

The first two weeks after implant are the most critical as far as activity restrictions. Depending on the dressing that was used at the implant, you may have to wait until your two-week follow-up appointment in the device clinic or your physician's office to have the dressing removed. If steri-strips are used without a waterproof dressing to cover them, by 1-2 weeks, they will begin to curl and fall off. It is best to allow them to fall off on their own. The healthcare provider you see at your two-week check will visualize the incision and area surrounding it looking for signs of infection. Redness, drainage, or warmth at the site of incision or if you develop a fever are all reasons to call your doctor as you may need to be seen earlier than the typical two-week follow-up. Also, if at any point you see your incision starting to open, let your physician's office know immediately. Many patients will have bruising and minimal swelling as they heal, and this is normal. Most will have the urge to itch the area as the tissue begins to heal on the inside giving that sensation. Do not itch the area.

Your physician will tell you his/her preferences on when you can resume driving and other typical activities of daily living. You will still need to be careful using the arm on the surgical side until at least 4-6 weeks post-implant. Do not make any jerking movements with that shoulder or arm as the more you stretch it above your head or behind your back, the more you pull on the leads and where they are implanted into the heart tissue. Even a minor amount of movement of the leads from where they were placed can cause major issues and possibly the need to revise the surgery to put the lead back where it belongs in the heart muscle. You don't want to completely immobilize your arm but it is better to be safe than sorry when it comes to even moderate stretching of that shoulder until 6 weeks post-op.

Your company representative may or may not discuss home monitoring with you at the time of implant. It is recommended that you utilize home monitoring for follow-up on the functioning of the device as well as basic information that will alert the physician if any harmful or potentially harmful situations are noted with your pacemaker. It is not required to utilize the home monitoring, and if it is your preference, you can always visit the clinic for in-person device checks two to four times per year depending on your device, the clinic's protocols, and the physician's preferences.

7

Device Interrogation

The device rep will check, or interrogate, your pacemaker the day after surgery with a computer called a programmer. A plastic device called a wand will be placed on your chest over the pacemaker, and it will "talk" to the pacemaker to receive a battery longevity estimation and information stored on the pacemaker. The information will be a record of any events (abnormal heart rhythms) since the implant. Also at that time, the device will be tested to ensure all parameters point to it working properly. This check will not hurt or bother you; most people can't even feel anything happening differently from what they have already been feeling since the device was implanted. One of the tests requires the tech to increase the heart rate of the patient by approximately 20 bpm. With new devices and patients who have not become accustomed to the way it feels to have the pacemaker make their heartbeat, they may be able to tell the difference. Some patients will feel dizzy or just uncomfortable if the increase in heart rate is too much for them. Also, patients with any type of heart block may also feel a bit dizzy or "woozy" if the tech allows their heart rate to go too low for too long. It is recommended the patient be sitting on the exam table with their back against the bed and feet up so if they do become dizzy or momentarily lose consciousness, they will be safer and less likely to fall down to the ground. Always let the representative, tech, or nurse controlling the programmer know if you are feeling dizzy or uncomfortable in any way during the interrogation.

The same type of check or interrogation will be performed at your two-week follow-up appointment as well as at six weeks and any time you come into the clinic for a pacemaker check thereafter. As mentioned above, your typical device follow-up schedule is twice a year in the device clinic. Even with home monitoring, it is necessary to come into the clinic for any programming changes needed to optimize your device and therapy.

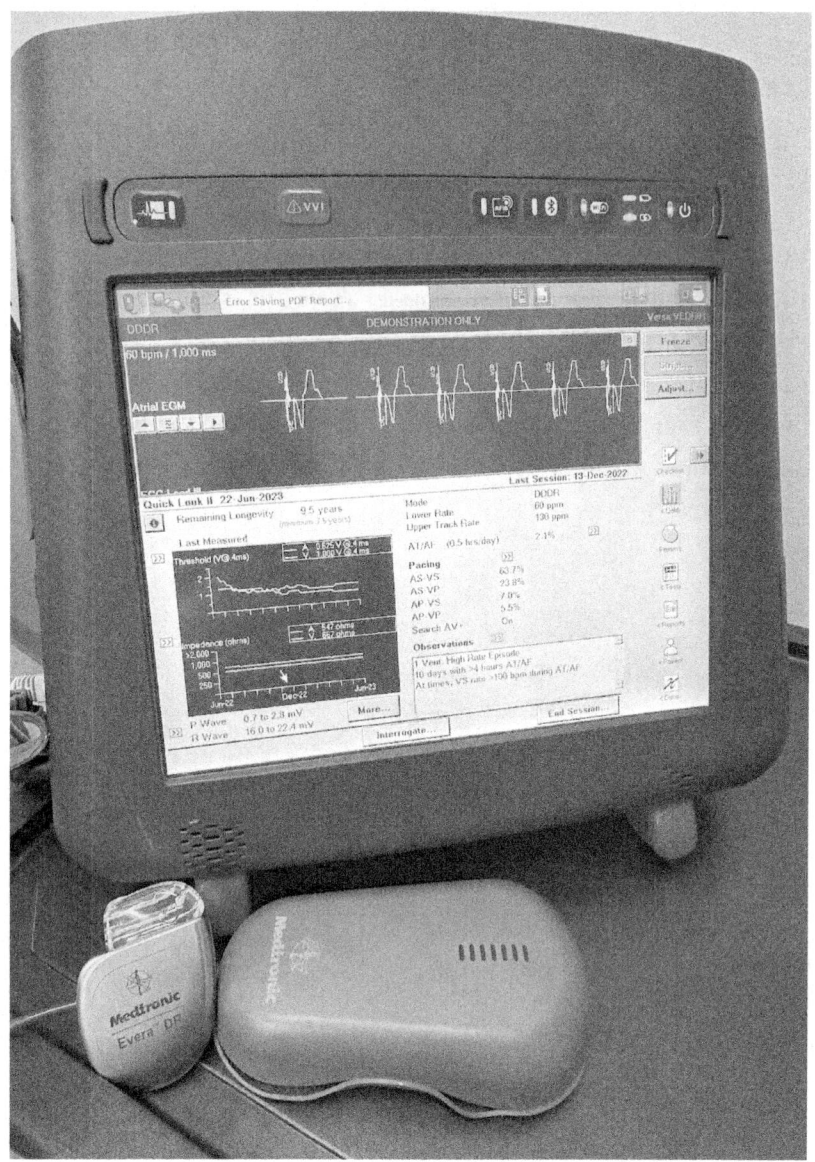

Bedside programmer used during interrogations

8

Living with a Pacemaker

The entire concept behind a pacemaker is to return to normal life without any loss of quality of life. The pacemaker is supposed to supplement the heartbeats your heart is unable to produce. Many patients will say they forget they have a pacemaker, and that's the way it should be. The pacemaker is meant to give you a quality of life you wouldn't otherwise have because you couldn't sustain normal activities without it.

You should be getting back to your usual, normal life and everyday activities by six weeks post-op. You can and are encouraged to be physically active. There are settings on the pacemaker that can help increase your heart rate with activity if your heart is not able to increase the rate on its own. You will have what is known as a low rate setting which tells the pacemaker when to start working or to make the heart beat if it senses your own heart rate fall below that setting. Usually, it is no lower than 60 bpm as a normal range for heart rate is 60 - 100 bpm.

If travel is your hobby, you will have no issues with planes, trains, or automobiles. You will go home with a paper ID card that shows information about your pacemaker, your doctor, and where your device was implanted. About 10 days after your surgery, you will receive a permanent ID card to replace that one. You should either carry that ID card with you or keep it in a safe place. Take it with you when you travel so you are able to show it when necessary, for example when you need to go through metal detectors. Let TSA agents know that you have a pacemaker. Also, take it with you when you see other healthcare professionals to make them aware that you have an implanted cardiac device. Most notably, dentists will need to know you have a pacemaker.

Avoid any machinery or electronic devices that have large magnets and thus magnetic fields. Microwaves and other household appliances, as well as small power tools, are all fine to use. Welding should be avoided. Cell phones should always be held on the side opposite the pacemaker and never carry your cell phone in a pocket directly over the pacemaker insertion site. Keep anything you know of that has any significant magnetic strength at least 6 inches away from your pacemaker.

*If you have a pacemaker, AVOID welding and keep magnets **at least 6 inches** away from your pacemaker!*

Continue taking all medications as prescribed by your physician. A pacemaker does not take the place of any of your heart medications but it works in conjunction with them to keep your heart beating at a regular, normal pace and in a regular rhythm. The pacemaker helps to control the electrical system of the heart, and has nothing to do with the vasculature or whether you can or will have a heart attack. It does not prevent heart disease or clogging of the arteries, therefore it does not prevent heart attacks.

9

Remote Monitoring

"Remote monitoring for cardiac implantable electronic devices is recommended by cardiology societies around the globe, including the European Society of Cardiology (ESC), Heart Rhythm Society in the US, and the Latin American Heart Rhythm Society, among others," (Biotronik 2022). As mentioned in the device interrogation section above, most implantable cardiac device companies offer home monitoring equipment. Each company's remote monitoring equipment is slightly different. Still, they all serve the same purpose: to reduce unnecessary in-clinic interrogations (for example, during the pandemic) but also to prevent adverse medical conditions from becoming unmanageable or from resulting in preventable death. The time between events and medical intervention is drastically reduced with the use of remote monitoring. In addition to detecting patient events that could lead to a detrimental outcome, home monitoring can also detect device malfunction, lead fracture, and battery depletion. It is also helpful in the early detection of arrhythmias such as atrial fibrillation which, undetected and untreated, could lead to stroke.

REMOTE MONITORING

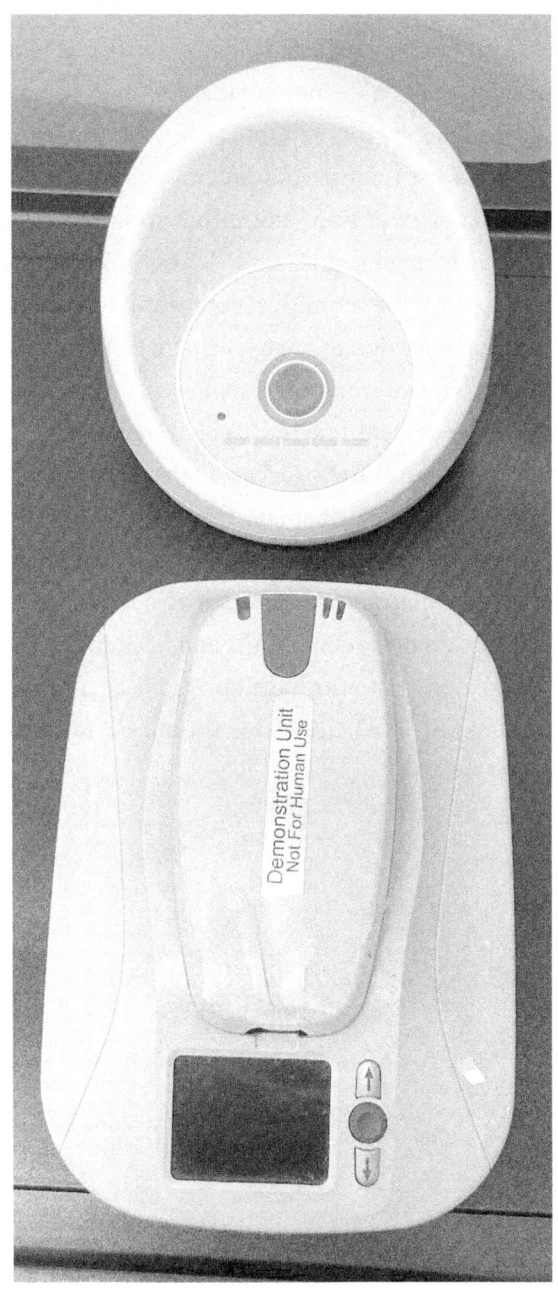

Examples of remote monitors

interested and keen to the idea of home monitoring. They have no qualms about using the remote monitoring equipment or even the more recently developed mobile phone applications that can be downloaded and used in place of the remote equipment. As opposed to equipment of the past, the majority of home monitors complete their daily and scheduled quarterly checks automatically without any involvement from the patient. Once the monitor is set up and functioning near the patient's bed, the patients don't have to participate in any other way with the transmissions. The information is sent via cellular networks and no longer needs wifi or a telephone line to be transmitted. Compared to only a few years ago, the entire process is fairly automated and should cause no further worries to the patient. However, older patients are still wary of the entire idea of an electronic device sitting by their bed to transmit device information to their clinic. Many would much prefer the human interaction of in-clinic visits and decline home monitoring altogether. Also, many patients have questions regarding the cost of home monitoring but those questions should be addressed by their insurance companies.

10

Conclusion

As a healthcare provider, it is my job to answer your questions to the best of my ability. As a device clinic nurse, I have found my patients are often confused and frustrated by how little they know about the device implanted in their chest. As a result of their confusion, many times they are also fearful of the device itself and how it will affect their daily lives. At the time of implant, lots of patients are worried that significant changes will have to be made to their lifestyles to accommodate their new device. Either too much was explained to them on the day of implant and they don't remember it or they have confused some of the information so they are under false assumptions. They come to the clinic overwhelmed. Ever since I have understood this and the answers to their questions, I have tried to ease their fears and help them understand as best I can. As all of my patients have one thing in common (an implanted cardiac device), they often have the same questions so I have contemplated making handouts to explain the most common questions and topics for quite some time. This book is my attempt to preempt the confusion and answer multiple questions in order to alleviate fear and worry. If you downloaded this book after your device was implanted, it is my prayer that you feel comforted knowing more and better understanding your new cardiac device and what to expect in the upcoming weeks, months, and years.

If I was successful in my mission to help you better understand your pacemaker, please do me a favor and leave a positive review for my book on Amazon. It will be much appreciated, and doing so will help others find the book more easily when they are in need.

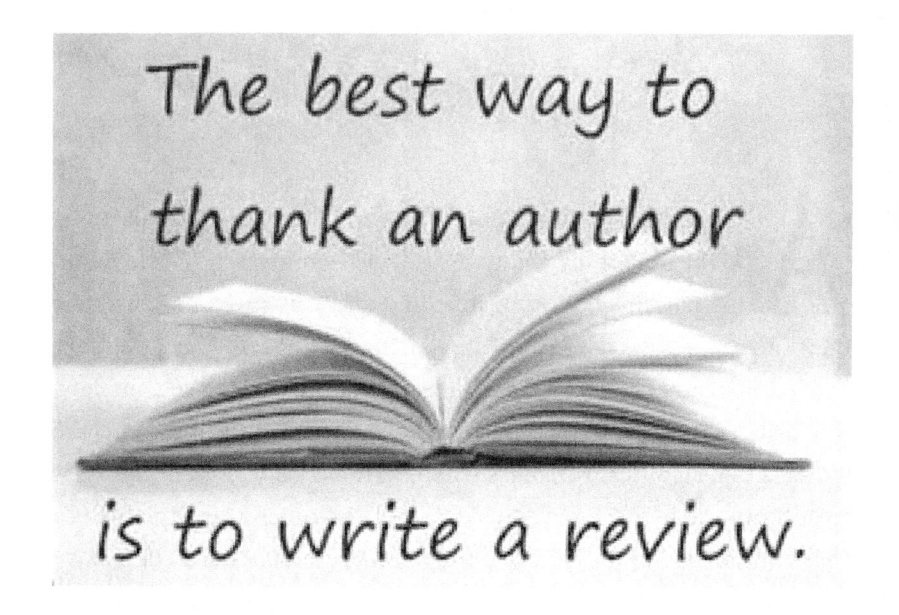

11

FAQs

As a device clinic nurse myself, I field many questions from patients every day. This book is a labor of love as I have always thought about compiling the repeated questions that my colleagues and I hear on a daily basis and distributing a FAQ sheet to patients when they are new to the implanted cardiac device clinic, sort of like part of a "welcome to the family" basket. Here is a list of those frequently asked questions that have not already been addressed in the previous chapters.

How long will the battery last?
Pacemaker batteries typically last between twelve and fifteen years but the longevity is based on how much it is used by the individual. The more pacing the individual requires, the less time it will take for the battery to be depleted.

What happens when the battery dies?
During the quarterly checks, one of the measurements we get is the battery longevity. Unless you do not keep up with your recommended check ups and you don't have a home monitor, your device clinic is

always aware of the amount of life your battery has left before it will need to be replaced. Your battery depletes like gas in your car's gas tank. When you are getting close to the end of the tank, the "gas" light comes on. In the world of pacemakers, that is called the device reaching ERI (elective replacement indicator) or RRT (recommended replacement time). It is at that time that your electrophysiologist will schedule you for your replacement surgery. As mentioned, ERI/RRT is the gas light; it means the battery then has 3-6 months left so it is time to get a new generator. The procedure for a generator change is less dangerous and less complex as long as you do not need any leads replaced. In that case, an incision is made in the same place as your original incision to visualize that generator. The leads are disconnected from the device, and a new device is connected to the leads before it is placed back in the same pocket, secured with a stitch and the incision reclosed. Downtime after the surgery is also not as long if the leads do not have to be replaced. Just about 2 weeks while the chest incision heals is normal.

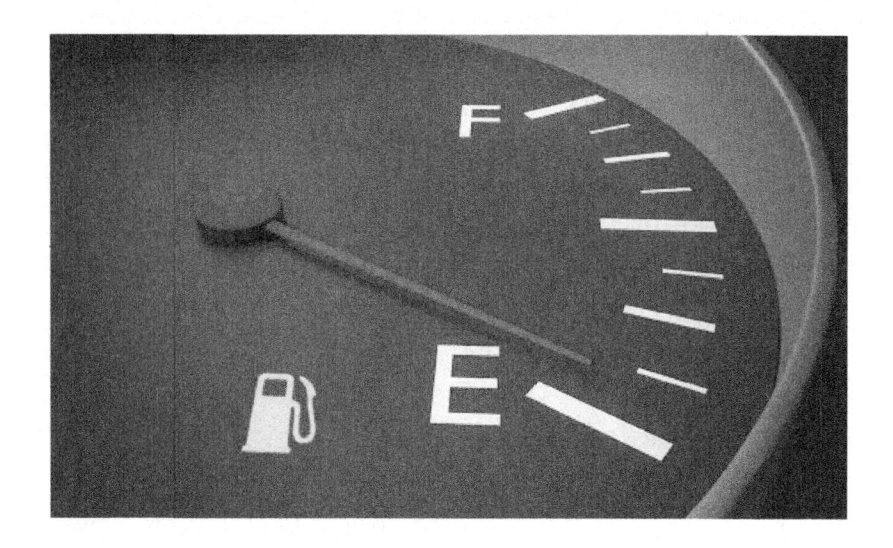

Can I have an MRI?

If your pacemaker is relatively new and both the generator and the leads are manufactured by the same company, chances are you will have no issues getting an MRI. However, what will happen is your doctor will have to send a request to the device clinic to have the staff review the safety of having an MRI with the device and leads (or system) you have implanted. When we receive a request, we check with the company regarding the safety of such a procedure. The MRI is a diagnostic machine that uses very large magnets to produce the images it produces, and the magnetic field of these magnets can sometimes affect the programming of the device in such a way (by electromagnetic interference) that it prevents effective pacing in situations when it is most definitely needed. An article published in a German medical journal explains probable reasoning for the death of 6 people in Germany in the 1980s who may have been the victims of ventricular fibrillation induced by asynchronous pacing which started during an unsupervised MRI procedure (Bovenschulte, et. al, 2012). Their devices' programming was affected/changed by the interference from the MRI. Thus, approval from the electrophysiologist for such a procedure and the research done before such a decision is made is essential to the safety of the patient who is in need of such a test.

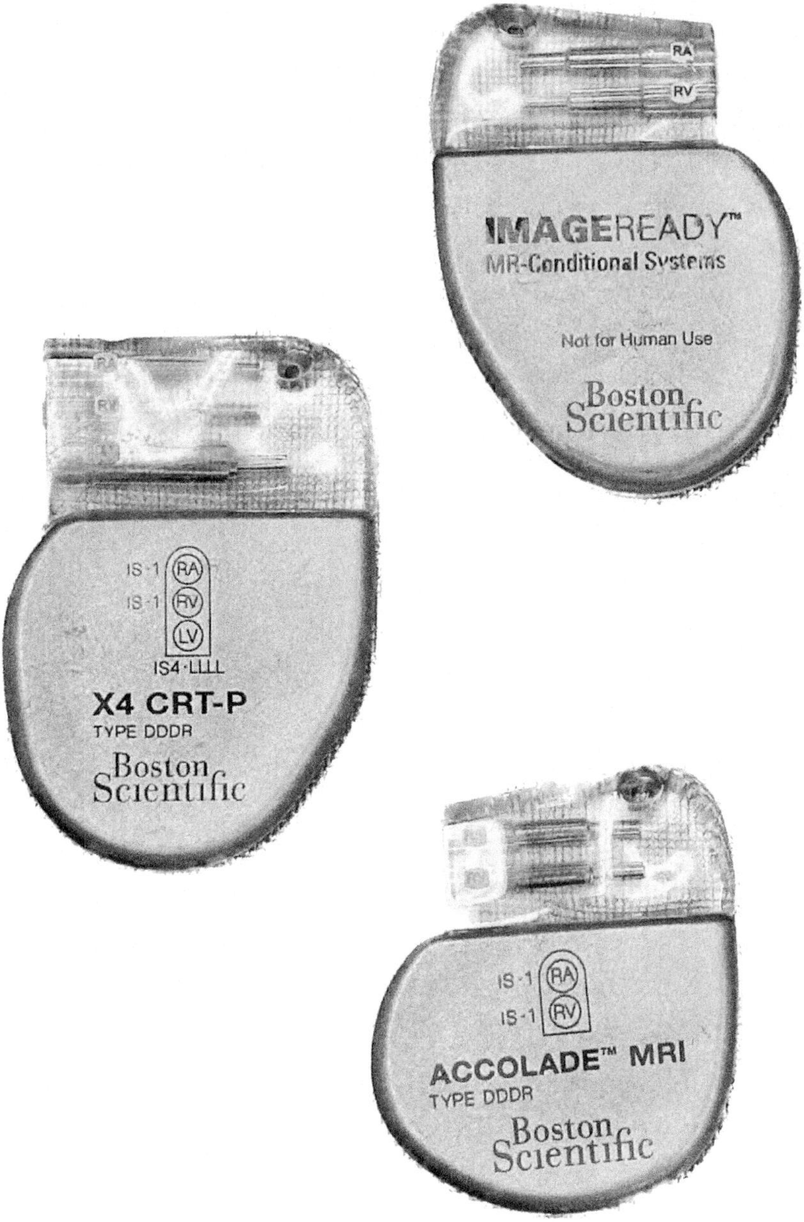
RA
RV
IMAGEREADY™
MR-Conditional Systems
Not for Human Use
Boston Scientific
IS-1 RA
IS-1 RV
LV
IS4-LLLL
X4 CRT-P
TYPE DDDR
Boston Scientific
IS-1 RA
IS-1 RV
ACCOLADE™ MRI
TYPE DDDR
Boston Scientific

12

References

Aquilina, O. (2006). A brief history of cardiac pacing. Images in Paediatric Cardiology, 8(2), 17-81. https://www.ncbi.nlm.nih.gov/pmc/articles/PMC3232561/

Biotronik (2022, November 28). Pandemic Sees Big Jump in Remote Monitoring Use, but Reimbursement Still a Barrier. News.Biotronik.com. Retrieved June 19, 2023, from https://news.biotronik.com/pandemic-sees-big-jump-in-remote-monitoring-use-but-reimbursement-still-a-barrier/

Bovenschulte, H., Schlüter-Brust, K., Liebig, T., Erdmann, E., Eysel, P., & Zobel, C. (2012). MRI in Patients With Pacemakers: Overview and Procedural Management. Deutsches Ärzteblatt International, 109(15), 270-275. https://doi.org/10.3238/arztebl.2012.0270

Dalia T, Amr BS. Pacemaker Indications. [Updated 2022 Aug 22]. In: StatPearls [Internet]. Treasure Island (FL): StatPearls Publishing; 2023 Jan-. Available from: https://www.ncbi.nlm.nih.gov/books/NBK507823/

Jeffrey, Kirk, and Parsonnet, Victor. "Cardiac Pacing, 1960–1985." *Circulation*, vol. 97, no. 19, 1998, pp. 1978–1991, https://doi.org/10.1161/01.cir.97.19.1978.

Madhavan M, Mulpuru S, McLeod C, et al. Advances and Future Directions in Cardiac Pacemakers. J Am Coll Cardiol. 2017 Jan, 69 (2) 211–235. https://doi.org/10.1016/j.jacc.2016.10.064

Morris, Thomas. [morrisngthomas].(2017, May 27). *Astonishingly, when Arne Larsson died in 2002 he had received twenty-two pacemakers in total, and outlived the surgeon who saved him.* [Image attached]. [Tweet]. Twitter. https://twitter.com/thomasngmorris/status/868427684489170945

van Hemel, N.M. and van der Wall, E.E. (2008). 8 October 1958, D Day for the implantable pacemaker. *Netherlands Heart Journal*, 16(Suppl 1), S3. https://www.ncbi.nlm.nih.gov/pmc/articles/PMC2572009/

Vandenberk, B., & Raj, S. R. (2022). Remote Patient Monitoring: What Have We Learned and Where Are We Going? Current Cardiovascular Risk Reports, 17(6), 103-115. https://doi.org/10.1007/s12170-023-00720-7

Varma N, Love C, Michalski J, et al. Alert-Based ICD Follow-Up. J Am Coll Cardiol EP. 2021 Aug, 7 (8) 976–987. https://doi.org/10.1016/j.jacep.2021.01.008

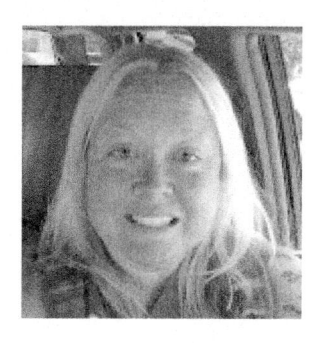

About the Author

I am a mom to two beautiful young men, Noah and Knox as well as my pups, Apollo and Gracie. I have been a registered nurse since January 2005, and I have been working as a device clinic nurse for 2 years. I also worked as a med-surge floor nurse, a surgical nurse and a mother/baby nurse. I enjoy going to the beach and drinking Sonic Oreo and Reese's Peanut Butter Master shakes (don't judge!)

Printed in Great Britain
by Amazon